T0193594

Cleo, I miss you babe. This pamphlet is in your memory. You will FOREVER be in my thoughts. You remain ALWAYS in my heart.

Love,

Shante'

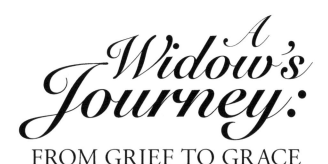

A Widow's Journey:

FROM GRIEF TO GRACE

Grieving My Spouse

REKESHIA S. HUDSON

WESTBOW
PRESS®
A DIVISION OF THOMAS NELSON
& ZONDERVAN

WestBow Press books may be ordered through booksellers or by contacting:

WestBow Press
A Division of Thomas Nelson & Zondervan
1663 Liberty Drive
Bloomington, IN 47403
www.westbowpress.com
844-714-3454

Scripture quotations marked (NLT) are taken from the Holy Bible, New Living Translation, copyright ©1996, 2004, 2015 by Tyndale House Foundation. Used by permission of Tyndale House Publishers, a Division of Tyndale House Ministries, Carol Stream, Illinois 60188. All rights reserved.

ISBN: 978-1-6642-3231-0 (sc)
ISBN: 978-1-6642-3230-3 (e)

Library of Congress Control Number: 2021908191

Print information available on the last page.

WestBow Press rev. date: 5/12/2021

Stages of Grief According to a Widow

Stages of grief are imperative to understand because navigating your emotions within this space may have you thinking you are crazy. You know, one moment you are glad, and the next moment you are angry and frustrated. My experience with grieving my husband can be compared to an ocean. Have you ever watched a beautiful blue ocean? One moment, there is peace. You may feel a slight breeze and hear the chirping of the birds. Abruptly, the waves may roar, causing the wind to become more forceful and powerful.

There have been encounters with grief while I am sitting at church, during a program at my daughters' school, and while in the middle of a phone call, just to name a few. I am including the five stages of grief, and along with that, I will transparently share my journey with grief during those stages. The sole purpose is to share with widows that what is felt is normal, and as long as you focus on healing, the grip from your hurt loosens.

1. Denial and isolation. Denial of anything is disbelief, which holds one in a dormant state. Think about a circumstance that triggered an initial response of denial. Were you in disbelief? Were you shocked? Were you stifled by what happened? The initial response to an unexpected situation is astonishment.

The death of my husband was so unexpected. My feelings of denial began at the moment I learned of his passing. I vividly remember hoping he was in the hospital and we could pray for him through his injuries. I remember verbally denying his death, even before I was told that he died. I recall thinking, *No, my husband is not dead.* Days, weeks, months, and even years later, I still deny that he is no longer here with me. Most days I look at pictures and with feelings of dejection, pinch myself or daydream only to discover this new normal is real. I sit in astonishment while contemplating on my husband, my soul mate, will never return to me on Earth.

I am in utter hurt and pain because what I continue to deny is my reality. Three years later, it still is true that he is not coming back to create the memories that we had planned. Denial is the state of avoiding what is true in order to prevent feelings that include hopelessness, anger, and hurt. My experience with denial was triggered when I thought about my new normal, which included growing old alone, raising my girls alone, and my girls being deprived of milestones experienced with their dad.

When I would look in the mirror, I would say repeatedly, "Cleo is dead. He is not coming back." By repeating this constantly, the reality of his absence settled in my mind, and while I was not okay with that idea, I had to begin to accept the truth. Denial of my loss did not make me feel better or feel as if he were still with me, but I was able to momentarily hide behind what I did not want to accept. It is comparable to someone trustworthy maliciously doing something towards you and you do not want to notice it.

There is not a time limit during this stage, but as each moment progressed, as I continued to traverse throughout this space solely, my denial became a reality, and no matter how much I did not want to accept the certainty of my loss, I began to confess what had taken place in my life. Have you ever wondered why a close friend became a distant friend, suddenly? Perhaps you reflected and presumed the distance was due to something you had done or said so you begin to replay your encounters?

Commonly, people go into isolation until they recover from situations. Isolation counteracts exposure of the emotion. It is a scapegoat from the world, support, and your community. Oftentimes, isolation is the answer to known problems that one is struggling to acknowledge or come to a solution for. My experience with isolation during the loss of my dear husband could be described as inactive and disinterested in personal endeavors.

During the first year as a widow, my focus was on surviving. More than anything, I was hoping to meet our basic needs. Along with widowhood came parenting alone. Survival was a must because parenting has always been a high priority. Even during the times that I isolated myself and withdrew myself from my loved ones, I had to survive in this lonely space that felt enclosed, scary, dark, and never-ending. I isolated myself from the joy that lay on the other side of my door, which was wives with husbands, children with fathers, hopeful futures, established, cheerful families, and joyful conversations with friends regarding careers, success, and their present day. I could not see past my agony.

Throughout this stage of isolation, I had no desire to be among the blessed ones, the successful ones. I was bitter, broken, confused, and almost lifeless. Sometimes I felt hopeful. Sometimes I feel hopeful. Sometimes I felt like I was going around in circles.

Throughout this period of denial and isolation, my support system did not leave me by myself, although they knew how I felt from me telling them and also from watching my changed behavior. During this phase of denial and isolation, I listened to my loved ones, although I did not always do what was suggested. I did not have the desire. My pain from my heartbreak had me crippled, halted, and yielded from the thought of progress. The greatest lesson from this stage that helped me was my isolation, but my loved ones did not disconnect from me. They knew the type of person I was before my loss, and they recognized my struggle to live. They were patient and prayerful during this stage of denial and isolation.

2. Anger. Anger is a responsive emotion towards something that offends you, hurts you, and changes your mood from positive to negative. Anger will cause headaches, back tension, stomach queasiness, and rage in your thoughts just to pinpoint. A few obvious responses. During the beginning stages of my grief, I expressed my anger towards my husband. I felt he had left me by myself to grow alone, to survive alone, to solve problems alone, and to raise our daughters alone. It was not his fault that he had suddenly left us.

Unconsciously, I would have toxic thinking that contributed to the fear of the future. I was furious when I saw husbands and wives. My love for couples had turned into a bitter and hopeless thought that led me to believe that after all the effort my husband and I had put into our marriage, it immediately ended. Talk about being upset at the world and my situation! I could not believe that we had followed the correct steps to life and—*boom!*—life forever changed.

To cope with my anger, I isolated myself perpetually because I did not want my fury to show while in public. Besides, I felt comforted being behind closed doors. Home was my safe place, my sanctuary, and I no longer had to face what was on the other side: cheer, hope, sunlight, two-parent households, children with fathers, dark nights, holding hands, and laughing. Routinely, I attended grief therapy, which permitted me to reminisce, cry, laugh, regain focus relative to the present, and rebuild my trust in living. It has taken years to fully become excited about living a wholesome life mentally. Present-day, I often find myself wondering if life will get better with someone or if I will remain in my singleness.

Currently, I am okay with the Lord's plan, but it has not always been this way. The idea of growing older alone has triggered frustration, fear, and anger. My husband and I married when I was twenty-three years old and he was approaching twenty-five years old. We grew up together, and the notion of living without him has crippled me like a sudden medical diagnosis changes the trajectory of one's future. My belief in love has always been powerful. I believe that love makes life possible, worth fighting for. When my first love left me, I just knew I would never be the same. I could not envision navigating this territory without the one who loved me through my good and through my bad.

3. Bargaining. Bargaining perpetuates vulnerability and blame, such that it overlays with anger. An example of bargaining would be saying, "If only I had taken him to work and picked him up that particular day, then things would have ended up differently." It is wishful thinking.

Bargaining takes place when you sit long enough while attempting to process, only to end up imagining what life would be like had you done something opposite of what you did. I mentally repeated, *What if I had called him sooner?* The truth is I will never know if that would have prevented my husband's death, no matter if I deem it would have or not. Bargaining is a form of mental distress. It traps your mind, disables proper thinking, and will keep you entangled if apt mental programming does not begin.

Whenever I began to bargain, I would allow the thought and then unpack it. By doing so, I was able to contemplate it until the end and attain an understanding that this circumstance was beyond my control and it has happened. There is no reverting.

Conceptually, I began to replace my negative with positive, good memories of my current situation, the time and health I have been given. The question persisted, "What will I do with the time afforded?" Do not allow mental defeat to rob you of any moments. If it comes, be resilient, be fierce, and affirm yourself.

4. Depression. The temperature outdoors was low, snow covered the bushes, and we had been at my mom's home for close to a month. The time had come to brave the other side of my mom's front door. My girls and I braved the crowd of the Civil Rights Museum as our first family outing without my husband. We did not attend alone. My cousins and their children joined us. As I write about that day, I recollect the picture that I posted on social media. It was the first picture I had posted since Cleo passed. Recounting the feeling that embraced my heart triggers my tears as I write. I felt depressed, sad, angry, dejected, furious, confused, and broken. Frequently,

I attempted to smile through the situation, but all I could think about was having to continue my life, adapt, look ahead, and live without my husband by my side. Needless to mention, I did not want to, but I knew I had to because of my daughters, if for no other reason. My husband would have been disappointed had I given up.

My emotions sparked whenever I would see a father and daughter or husband and wife. Sentiments of bitterness and anxiety overwhelmed my spirit most days early on. This was certainly due to the hurt residing within my heart, the fear of living alone and raising my daughters without my husband,

and the feeling of no longer overcoming the odds. Undoubtedly, I never wanted to rear my daughters in a single-parent household because that is how I grew up, and I neglected so much that it has been a goal to attain self-assurance, family oriented activities such as vacations, game night, dinner around the table, within my adulthood and throughout parenthood.

Fortunately, during this stage, I remained resilient, and though sorely depressed, I managed to remain in counseling and learn coping mechanisms to apply to my unexpected moods that I could control, such as my thoughts that embraced weariness and hopelessness. I combated those thoughts with prayer, writing, affirmations, and talking with a trusted friend. Expressions of irritability were managed by deep breathing, calling my name, and relaxing my shoulders while reciting an affirmation, such as "For I can do everything through Christ, who gives me strength" (Philippians 4:13).

There are levels of depression, and being aware of that, I knew I did not want to fall deep into the pit of major depression. I did not want my situational depression to turn into repetitive days of gloom, inability to get out of bed, a day without upkeep, isolation from loved ones, and withdrawal from everything that required verbal communication rather through text, email, or social media. Deliberately, no matter how horrible I felt, I managed to express my feelings to someone or something. Perpetually, I connected to my new reality by saying, "He's not coming back, Rekeshia. He's not coming back." I had to internalize that fact by constantly saying so in the mirror. It pained me more and more, but I was grasping what was true rather than rejecting it. I would cry, inhale, and exhale, as strange as that seems, as I continued to recite, "He's not coming back, Rekeshia."

Now, am I saying that prevented the pit of depression? Well, not solely, but partially. My mind was training to accept what had become normal: living without my husband, traversing parenting alone, living in this huge world, and making decisions without my backbone. Through this mental training, I began to believe what was true, and along with therapy, I could clearly envision my ability to live peacefully and fearfully, even if it meant with a broken heart.

In some cases, depression inflicts feelings of worthlessness, lowered self-esteem, uncertainty, deranged life perspective, and lack of interest. My advice includes paying attention to your body's changes and knowing what triggers your emotions. If adverse feelings persist, it is a healthy idea to seek a medical professional.

Grief is sneaky, and unexpectedly, sadness may turn into a major depression. However, I am proof of what does not have to occur, even under the circumstance.

5. Acceptance. During the stage of depression, I began to recite, "He's not coming back, Rekeshia." Not only did this recitation connect me to what was true, but it positioned my heart to begin to accept the absence of my husband. As days progressed, I knew it was true. I grounded myself in that thought so that I would, with all five senses, be in touch with my new reality. I had dodged the truth for so long, but I had to be honest in order to move forward. I had to face reality in order to take the next step, which for me was being intentional, beginning again rather than only surviving.

Growing in God and Goodness

Annually, my uncle celebrates his birthday with a bash where friends and family are invited to dance and eat a variety of food. In January 2019, I recall dancing to every upbeat song that the deejay blasted through the sound system. Vividly, I am reminded of the adrenaline rushing throughout my body while dancing with Cleo as I closed my eyes and reminisced of old times when he would take me dancing because he knew I enjoyed dancing so much.

That feeling of nostalgia filled my heart with reflection, gratitude, pain, regret, liberation—just a mix of emotions. However, the more I embraced my feelings, the closer I became to walking in acceptance and growing in my healing.

In October 2019, I encountered a turning point in my life. Before October 2019, I was in sole survival mode. I remained disinterested in anything pertaining to self-image and self-improvement. Throughout these feelings of despair, I did nevertheless continue to connect to the ministry through my church, attend counseling, and hang out with my friends when I felt up to doing so. It was seldom. I was honestly going through the motions. I did my best to fight feelings of hopelessness and toxic thoughts of uncertainty about my future love life. I was physically present but mentally drained and depressed.

But one weekend, God used someone to show me the possibility of living in the fullness of joy, loving wholeheartedly and fearlessly, and laughing until my belly aches. My deliverance began.

From October 2019 until the present day, it has been a bit wavering, but my mind has been more stable than it was in December 2017. Growing in God was at the forefront of my mind, but I was inconsistent in my study time and in my prayer life. I lived with so much bitterness and pain.

As time progressed, the Lord continued to nudge me by His Word being preached through my pastor, by centering me around God-fearing women, and by continuously allowing me to wake up to care for my greatest blessing besides my salvation: my two God-given miracles who are my daughters. My relationship with God helped me to fight for my sanity and regain my desire to live relentlessly. Not only to fulfill my calling but because I knew my daughters could feel my spirit, whether it was negative or positive. The girls deserved a vibrant, joy-filled parent considering all the unexpected hurt they have had to endure. Undoubtedly, God continues to carry me every step of the way.

Once I was restored with peace and a definite decision to live a purpose-driven and happy life, I began to focus on healthy ways to revive my spirit. There were mental battles, which is why constantly praying and talking to trustworthy friends remained imperative.

Additionally, practices that I use with my daughters and myself include reciting daily affirmations, engaging in art therapy, deep breathing, and meditation. We are connected to a Bible-believing church. My girls are linked to a healthy learning environment and love to attend school, which has served as a safe haven for them to learn, be loved, and be expressive. We attend family dinners. We frequently count our blessings because we believe that an attitude of gratitude keeps us living in the moment and less stressed. There are reasons to fret and be furious, but we choose to stay in a space of gratefulness.

It is easy to be robbed of the present moment by moping and regretfully thinking about things out of your control. There lies so much peace in a space of gratitude. What you focus on consumes you and dictates your mood. Arriving and growing in God does not mean my grief has disappeared, but it is managed more healthily. I grieve my husband with hope for my present and with belief that I am capable of raising respectful and kind daughters. The advantage in life is we are afforded choices and decisions.

As I continued to grow in God by reading my bible more and showing goodness towards others, which is what I love, I could feel myself living life on purpose. Through this process, I was training my mind to focus on life in the present and do what mattered and what was within my ability momentarily. In my opinion, moment by moment is how life should be lived, allowing goals to be guides but always remembering to live intentionally.

Soak it all up, feel with all your heart, and use all five senses. Every instant is indeed a gift to develop in God and extend goodness. An attitude of gratitude is a transformational regimen to begin the day. What comes from the heart reaches the heart. Allowing the blue skies in and the gray skies out has positioned me to wake up to new mercies willingly, an opportunity to walk in grace, fulfill a life destined for purpose, live abundantly by faith, and unapologetically evolve into who I am supposed to become. Life as I know it has met me with countless punches, but I am still standing.

This one thing I know fiercely is "I press on to reach the end of the race and receive the heavenly prize for which God, through Christ Jesus, is calling us" (Philippians 3:14).

"The LORD will send rain at the proper time from his rich treasury in the heavens and will bless all the work you do. You will lend to many nations, but you will never need to borrow from them" (Deuteronomy 28:12). Amid life's challenges, God has His hands on me and continues to use me for the purposes of building His kingdom, by helping those who are despondent and visually impaired by their current state in life. I am a testimony of living with a repaired heart. Restoration takes effort, but it is attainable.

Talk with a professional, remain prayerful for healthy direction, put a plan in place, and execute the plan. Your heart will beat normally again. Your ears will be in tune with the sounds of life again. You will not always feel this way. Do not give up the fight. Choose to grow in God and show goodness towards others.

Growing in Grace

Grace is the favor shown by God not because of one's deeds but because of His love and care. For example, when my girls arrive home on Wednesdays, they are greeted with fresh flowers, not because of a good deed they have performed but because of the love I want to express toward them. Grace is like the "just because" gifts given from loved ones. Whenever you think of "just because," revert to GRACE: **G**od's **R**iches **A**t **C**hrist's **E**xpense. Each morning you wake up is another gift of GRACE.

Throughout my new normal, I learned to adapt to navigating life alone. Through grace and vision, I subscribed to WordPress in April 2020 out of obedience to my Creator. However, I did not publish my first blog post until August 2020. As mentioned, temptation invites itself, hindering me from clearly hearing and preventing me from writing what I know to be true and life changing for myself and others.

In September 2020, I launched my foundation in memory of my husband to serve as a legacy for my children and those who knew him. Additionally, I have united with a few widows who have allowed me to walk through their journey of widowhood. It is one thing to search the internet for resources that will support your dejected state of mind, but it means so much more when you are supported by someone who has been living what you newly experience. My experience has been purpose driven and humbling, and it keeps me in a space of gratitude.

As I grow in grace, it is my prayer that wherever you are in this walk, whether it is one day, one week, one month, one year, or fifty years, the love for your spouse may never fade, and that is the goal, but you get to decide to live a despondent lifestyle filled with melancholy and slothfulness or grow in grace in the midst of grit and live a purpose-driven life full of memories and a multitude of joy.

The following are a few affirmations that are accessible in my memory bank:

- I am healed. _____

- I am loved. _____

- I am brave. _____

- I am patient. _____

- I am forgiving. _____

- I am purposeful. _____

- I will live out each moment in the _____

  moment. _____

- I am enough. _____

- I've got this. _____

Grief is like an ocean filled with waves—some gentle and some more boisterous. Waves are certainly unpredictable. Because you can't time what may trigger your emotion, it is so important to access tools in what I call a mental toolkit. A few tools in my toolkit include

- Prayer _____
- Grief counseling _____
- Support from friends _____
- Volunteering _____
- Release through tears _____
- Art therapy coloring books _____
- Completing crossword puzzles _____
- Reading scriptures and self-help books
- Affirmations _____
- Working out _____

No matter if the loss of your spouse was unexpected or you were conditioned to prepare, the pain of losing a spouse, someone you shared your space with, does not change that fact. I remember feeling uncovered, meaning my husband, the head of my household, was no longer here to protect me. The lack of security lingered for quite a while and still is present in moments when I am out alone. I recall feeling as if no one would be to the rescue in the event of unforeseen and uninvited happenings. There were some things only he understood. There were some things only he would agree upon. Feelings of despair invaded my space and clouded my way. No matter how I maneuvered to position myself to attain consistency within my emotions and within my safety, emptiness resided.

It took a lot of work to arrive where I am mentally today. It took a made-up mind to reach this point. Even when I made up my mind, I wavered. Through my wavering, I still committed myself to implement the work to stabilize my mind and emotions so that I could live a life not free from grief but free from the bondage that grief upheld. I wanted to prevail over my circumstance. I wanted to be constant in my life choices. Today, I can say that I am not where I would have imagined three years ago, but I have an expectant heart and my life is full of possibilities. Guess what? So is yours! Live life on purpose in purpose.

Printed in the United States
by Baker & Taylor Publisher Services